THE HEALING POWER OF

NATURAL ANTIBIOTICS

Detailed guide on how to Purchase the Healing Power of Natural Antibiotics Legally & Cheap; without Doctor's Prescription

By

Doctor Eliza parker

TABLE OF CONTENT

CHAPTER ONE

INTRODUCTION TO ANTIBIOTICS

The killing and inhibiting of bacteria growth is with the help of Natural Antibiotics

Some people thought antibiotics are modern medicine; the truth is that it has been existing since several centuries. Natural Antibiotics as many people know are gotten from natural sources.

It is noted that since drug based antibiotics came into existence, natural antibiotic have been left to seat behind.

It was recently noted that drug based antibiotic have huge side effects and it is regularly demanded in a high rate. Your digestive system is affected anytime you take in a drug based antibiotic thereby affecting the bacteria that are healthy in your gut. These can cause the following to your body:

- ❖ Your immune system will be weakened
- ❖ Disease related to gut will be contacted. example is crohns

❖ **Deficiency in some nutrient**

The guts that are affected by these drug-antibiotics are damaged in less than few weeks. The more you continue taking this prescribed antibiotics the more your body damages along side with it

From findings, it is noted that every three person, one is given to take antibiotics even if it is not needed by that person's body. The misused of this antibiotic drug to anybody and has made bacteria and antibiotic resistant to be formed and scientist have not be able to fight it out.

The main point here is that drug-antibiotics are causing more harm to good due to its side effects

Natural antibiotic are chemical preserved free and cause no harm to our body.

Below is the list of antibiotics that you can use at home with full assurance of its medicinal content.

CHAPTER TWO

MANUKA HONEY

This is assign as the most special and beneficiary kind of honey that is used today on planet. It has many health benefits to man among which are greater infection fighting quality.

Manuka honey differs from other honey because it is developed from bee that is pollinated with manuka bush.

Research has proven that manuka honey contains these following substances: Hydrogen peroxide, dihydroxyacetane and methylglyoxal. These three main substance is what makes it possible for manuka honey to has potent antimicrobial properties.

It also discovered from studies that Staph infections can be kill with the use of manuka honey.

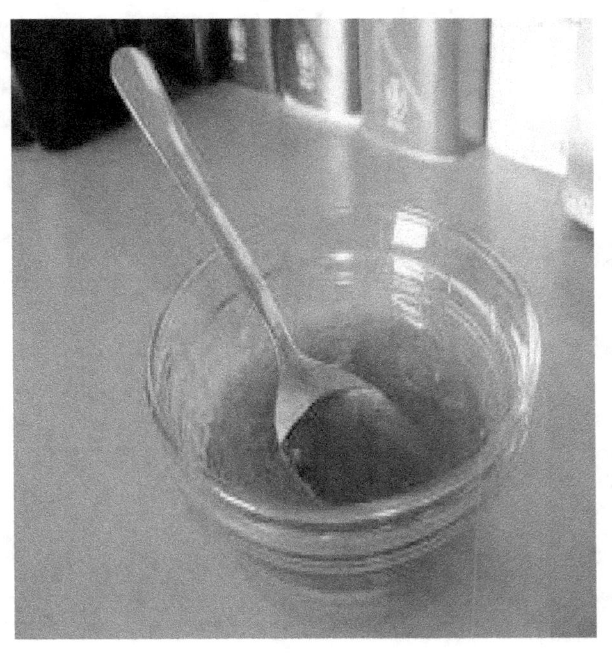

BEST GUIDE ON HOW TO USE MANUKA HONEY.

- ✓ When you have skin or oral infections,what manuka honey will do is to help fight that bateria and boost your immune system.

  It is used on the top surface of your skin and can also be eaten since it is sweet so as to boost your immune.

It is one of the approved way to fight bacteria.
The affected area of your skins should get manuka honey content on it,cover with a band aid.

HOW TO RECOMMEND MANUKA HONEY

If neighbor or friends around you are caught with cold or are not too healthy,I recommend that a tea spoon full be taken so as to prevent and treat such illness.

To make manuka honey more effective in treatment and prevention, mix manuka honey with cinnamon and ginger. it is also recommended that you take manuka honey once daily for longer healthy life style but considering it cost, it might not be possible daily

HOW TO BUY AND KNOW BETTER MANUKA HONEY

Manuka honey is available as any other supplement in the market. it has a range of different quality and very expensive. Because it is expensive try and get a better one that has high potency.

<u>NOTE</u>: when your immune system is not in support of taking manuka honey,try and avoid it unless prescribed medically.

CHAPTER THREE

A.OREGANO OIL

This oregano oil can not be compare as the herb you will like to appy to your meal called pasta sauce. comparing it with manuka honey,it is more medicinal than food because it contain distilled extract from medicinal grade oregano.

Carvacrol and thymol are the two main potent content of oregano oil. These two content can powerfully fight different grade of pathogens which are known as harmful microbes.

Example like carvacrol can fight a great range of antimicrobial effects. Several researches has proven that oregano can treat the following diseases:

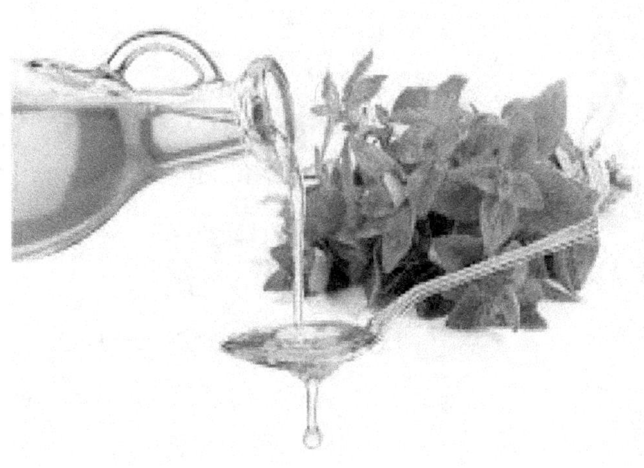

1. FUNGAL INFECTION, example is thrush which is formed or originated by candida.

2. BACTERIAL INFECTIONS

3. PARASITES

4. VIRUSES

5. INFLAMMATION

6. ALLERGIES

On the planet today, it is known that oregano oil is one and only best natural antibiotics. It is noted that several illness has been treated with oregano oil among which are:

- ✓ Yeast infections

- ✓ Foot or nail fungus

- ✓ Sinus infections

GENERAL USES OF OREGANO OIL

Different infections show different approach on how the oil will be used.

FOOT OR NAIL FUNGUS

It is recommended that a teaspoon full of oregano oil

is put in a water container and soak your feet inside the container. you might also wish to dilute the oil by collecting one drop of oregano oil mixing together with a well measured teaspoonfull of olive oil content. At the stage, you can apply put it on your skin or nail

SINUS INFECTION

Get a pot of water that is at its steaming point ,add few drops of oregano oil to it, next is for you to take in breath of the steam. Take proper care while breathing

in the steam because it is
very hot.

<u>ORAL INFECTIONS LIKE
THRUSH</u>

You will have to get a drop of
oregano oil + a teaspoon full
of cold coconut oil. Put it in
the mouth and wait for a few
minute and later rinse it out.
Carry out this task for 3 times
or make it 4 times daily.

How to Buy and Know Better Oregano Oil.

Since pesticide
contamination are
possible, it is preferred

that you get the best oregano species. Origanum Vulgare and Thymus Capitatus are the main content content that make oregano oil special. You must make sure that at least one of these best species must be available before you purchase it.

<u>NOTE</u>: you must not use this oregano oil internally so as not to destroy or kill some vital bacteria that are in your gut

CHAPTER FOUR

GARLIC (EXTRACT)

Garlic is known to be a delicious vegetable that most persons add to their meal. It is far more than that because it has an additional important as a powerful antibiotic that has been well tested . It is found that garlic has an active substance known as Diallyl sulphide and it is more effective than many other antibiotics. Some infections that garlic can fight are:

✓ Parasites

✓ Bacteria

✓ Viruses

✓ Fungi

Garlic functions in two ways which are the killing of infection and also the building of my immune system.

Research has show that a daily usage of garlic will help avert cold and it symptoms with a percentage rate of 63% to 70%. Garlic has other health benefits outside the listed above benefits;

- ❖ It helps to boost cholesterol level

- ❖ It lowers blood pressure

- ❖ It helps boost athletic activities.

- ❖ It help treat ear infection

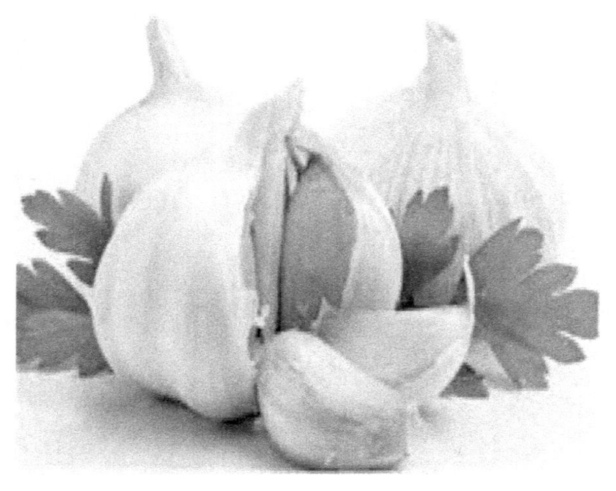

GENERAL USES OF GARLIC

It is known that most person add garlic to their food so as to have a good smell out of it. It is advice that for it to be used medically to treat an infection, it needs to be taken raw because that is when the antibiotic content will still be active. Drying and cooking will help to lose it medical content.

HANDLING SKIN INFECTION

One teaspoon cold compressed olive oil + one clove of crushed garlic.

Put the garlic in the olive oil and let it remain there for 30minutes then strain it. You can place it in warm water if you want the water warm and then apply some few drop to the area that is affected.

HANDLING EAR INFECTION

Garlic infused oil can be used to treat ear infection. Just collect small quantity of the oil which must be warm and then apply to the spot or part affected in the ear which should be done hourly. Ear wax built in the ear will also be loosen when applied.

HANDLING BOOSTING OF IMMUNE SYSTEM.

All you need to do is crushing one clove of garlic because chewing it might not be too easy and scare friend away due to its choking smell. The crushed garlic should be swallowed at least once per day and then your immune system is set for boosting.

How to Buy and Know Better Garlic.

Try and make sure that you get a better garlic that are original and not from china. Your garlic must be organic in nature

same as when selecting
the oil.

CHAPTER FIVE

B. CINNAMON

Cinnamon has been known as one of the widest most used spice.it is known as a fighter of a wider range of dangerious bacteria and fungal infection. Cinnamon has an inbuilt quality of inhibiting the growth and mycotox in the production of certain fungi. In details,cinnamon helps to kill all fungal infection and help to stop it from forming any compound that can cause tissue damage.

Here are cinnamon medicinal advantage and its ability to treat the following:

> Help in treating oral infections and bad breath.

> Help to treat gut discomfort.

> Help to treat acne that are mainly caused by bacteria.

➢ Help to treat Hemorrhaging

Cinnamon has nothing bad in it rather it is more loaded with delicious healthy benefit.

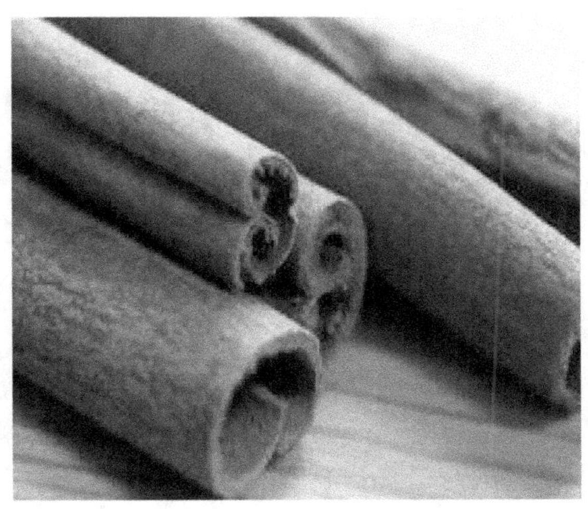

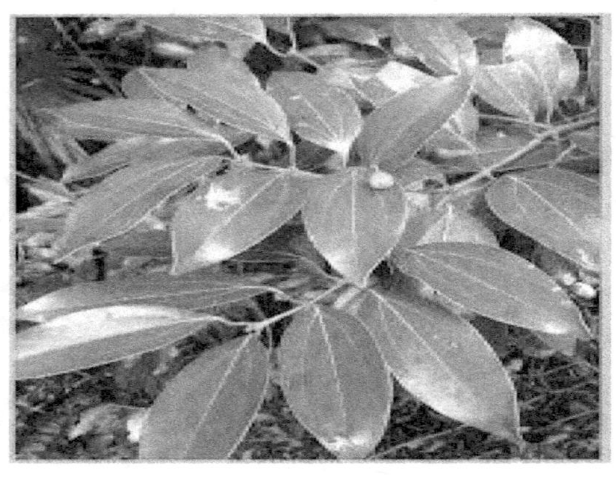

GENERAL USE OF CINNAMON

It is use as internal booster with powder, as external with oil.

Cinnamon is best used together with other natural antibiotics. It is the location of an infection that tells you will apply the medication.

<u>HANDLING SKIN INFECTION</u>

A few drop of Ceylon cinnamon of high quality is mix together with manuka honey. This mixture is applied on the surface of the affected area. This work very well and faster since it is a combination of two different   natural antibiotics.

HANDLING INTERNAL INFECTION

Get high quality of ceylon cinnamon powder together with manuka honey or raw organic honey. This mixture is taken twice daily for the prevention of cold and from getting sick

HOW TO BUY AND KNOW CINNAMON OIL

The Ceylon cinnamon you must buy must be organic type. it can be used for medicinal purposes or spice. Most cinnamon that is sold in several stores contains high quantity of coumarin which has toxin content in it that can destroy your liver. The organic Ceylon cinnamon might not be seen locally rather

make proper research
about it up to online
search.

CHAPTER SIX

GINGER

Ginger is another well known antibiotics that has natural compound as its content. Those natural content can do the following:

- ✓ Help soothe issue of discomfort and digestion.
- ✓ Help destroy infections
- ✓ Help reduce inflammation
- ✓ Help relieve nausea
- ✓ Help increase stomach acid so as to calm digestion after every meal. It is adviced that raw ginger be served with raw foods as to help in the prevention of

foodborne illness. Ginger should also be taken raw as garlic so as to benefits its antibiotic effects.

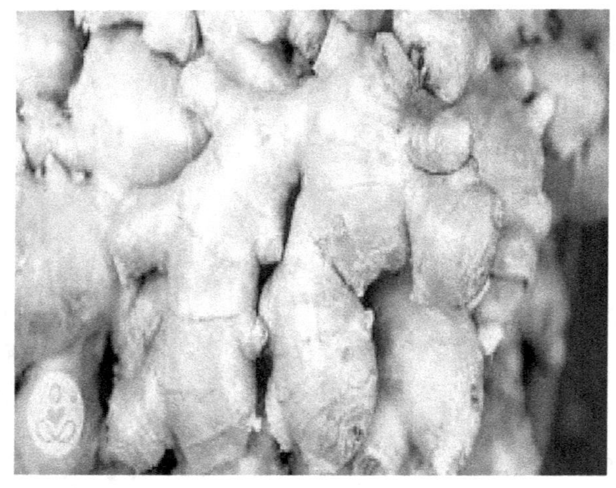

GENERAL USES OF GINGER

It is advised that ginger should be combined with other antibiotics for potent effectiveness, general health and immune booster. Example is the combination of raw ginger, raw honey and cinnamon to destroy Flu. Eaten ginger ordinarily is not as easy but with combination to other antibiotics makes it better in taste. Ginger is advice to be used internally only and not on the skin because it is irritating.

HOW TO BUY AND KNOW GINGER

Visit any store closer to you and get organic ginger. If you have any excess of it, store it in your freezer. The ginger can be grated with a grater and use for salad dressings or an inspired Asian dishes. If you cannot use it raw, cook it slightly. The benefits of ginger is gotten from its ginger extract pills and ginger candy.

CHAPTER SEVEN

PAUD' ARCO

Paud' Arco is a rain forest tree back which is very medicinal and very common in South America. Below are some of its assistance to health.

> Fever
> Candida overgrowth
> Ulcers
> Chronic inflammation

Paud'Arco is very active in the fight against Viral, Fungal and bacterial infections. Some researcher discover that beta-lapachone is the cause of antimicrobial effects. This lapachone helps to prevent replication of viruses and kills bacteria by inputting cellular respiration. Paud' Arco is the best assign herbs that can fight candida overgrowth in the gut.

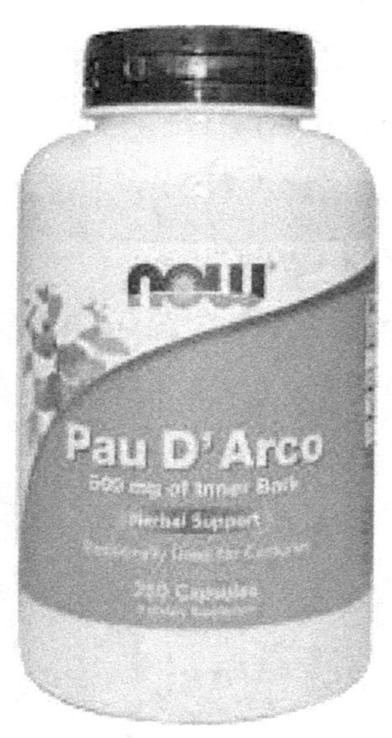

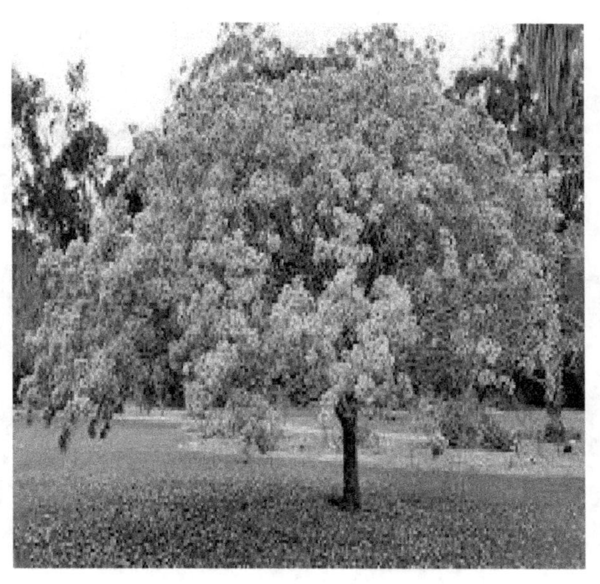

GENERAL USES OF PAUD' ARCO

Paud'Arco can be used both internally with tablet and externally with tincture. Some person don't always take the correct doses so it is advice that you use it for oral and skin infection purposes. It works perfectly for oral candida(thrush),sore throat and skin care.

It is not recommended for children and always ask permission from a health expert before taking any of these natural medication.

HOW TO BUY AND KNOW PAUD' ARCO

PAUD' ARCO can be in form of tea ,tablet or tincture form.

Don't go for the tea form since it don't dissolve in water.it is recommended that you go for the tincture or tablet with the instruction written on it.

THE END